Rocklocomotion

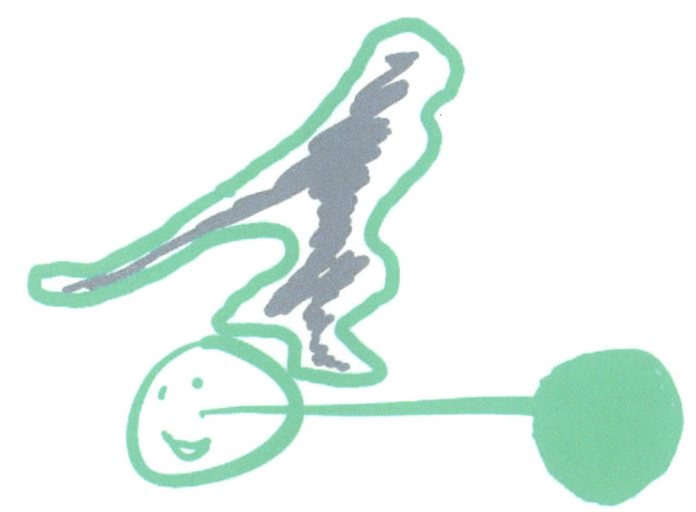

by

Dan Furlong

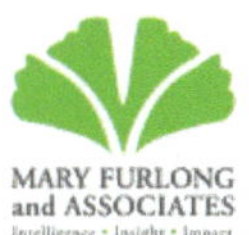

www.rocklocomotion.com

Rocklocomotion

By

Dan Furlong

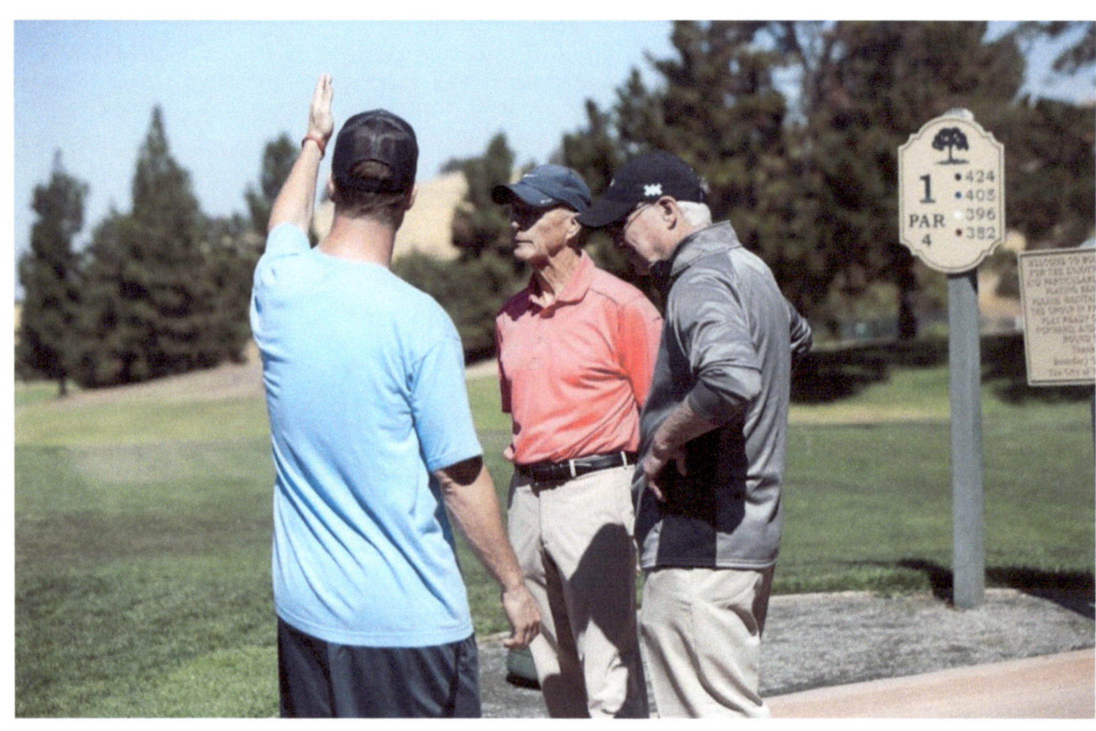

TABLE OF CONTENTS

Get in the right locomotion mindset - 3

Find a healthy locomotion hero - 4

Stay sharp and involved - 6

Learn your rights - 6

Consider moving to a community supporting a

healthy locomotion lifestyle - 11

Use technology to help you move - 14

Appreciate your body - 30

Roll Hard - 33

- Glendale Rough Riders - 34

The Rocklocomotion Menu - 34

Rocklocomotion

- Get in the right healthy locomotion mindset-

Be kind to yourself:

Be kind to yourself.

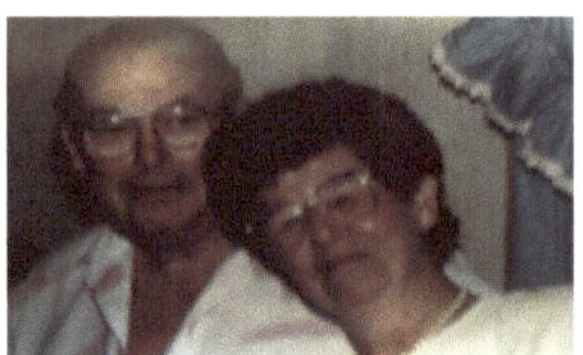

Dan & Cele Simpson

Put on some music:

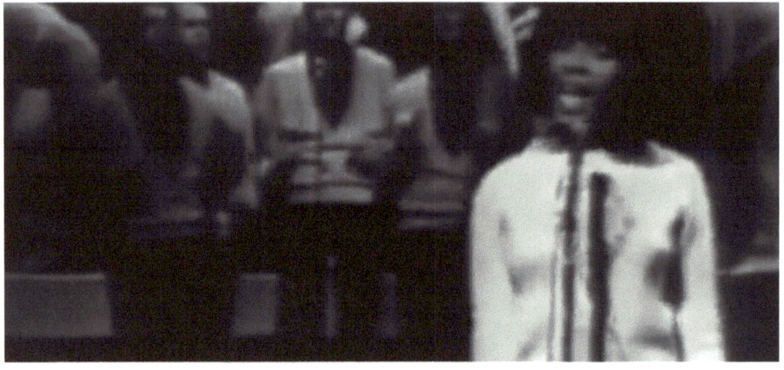

Little Eva

Watch a movie. Movies are magic. Relax. Tell someone a joke.

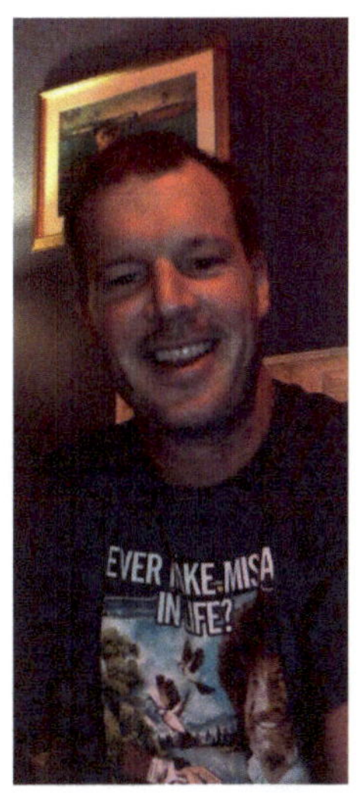

- **Find a healthy locomotion hero** -

We are better than we think, and we need to give ourselves more [credit](). This does not necessarily mean spoiling yourself, though that can be a [good way to start]().

Finding a way to stay mobile is an important part of living a fully self-actualized life. This does not, necessarily, mean physically moving.

Stephen Hawking was one of the most influential human beings the planet will ever see.

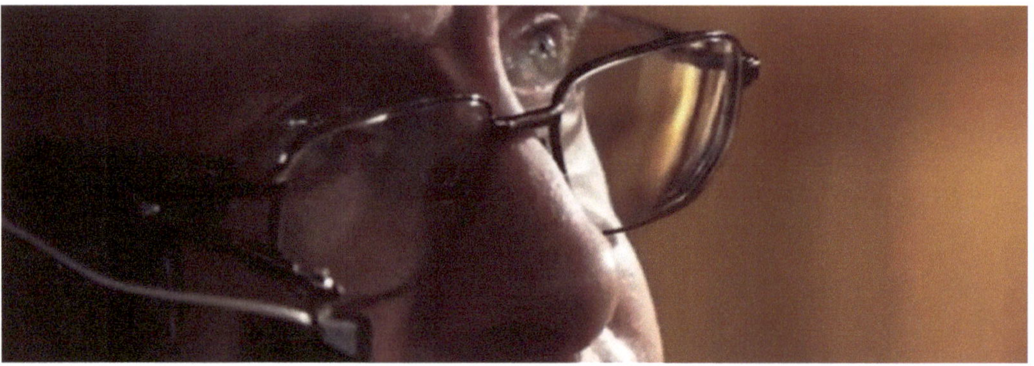

As a vibrant and brilliant young man, Stephen was diagnosed with Lou Gehrig's disease. The disease left his mobility impaired. However, Stephen's mind was free to contemplate the mysteries of the universe. He blessed humanity with countless brilliant observations and theories, and made cosmology understandable to the masses.

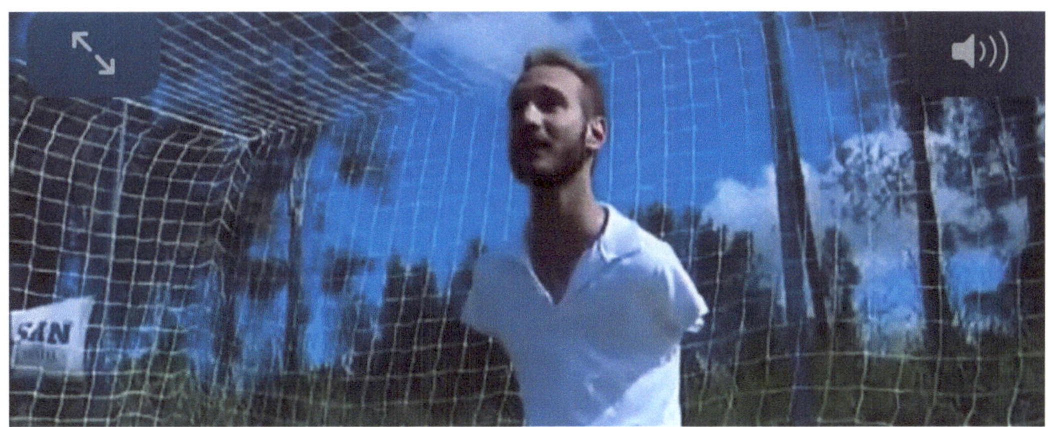

Nicholas James Vujicic

People like Nicholas James Vujicic, an inspirational speaker, and athlete with an incredible spirit; and [Josh Burger](), a disability advocate and all-around incredible person, show us that that we have limitless potential.

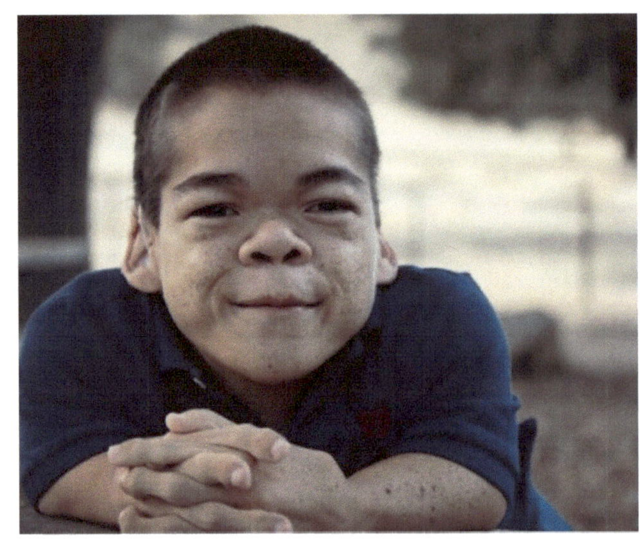

Josh Burger

Athletes like 4 time Canadian Wheelchair Tennis Champion and Paralympian Joel Dembe, show us that we can be empowered, thrive and have a full life, through our independence.

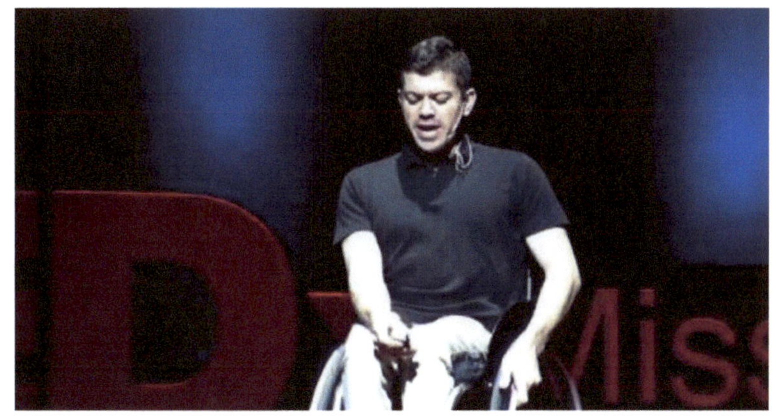

Joel Dembe

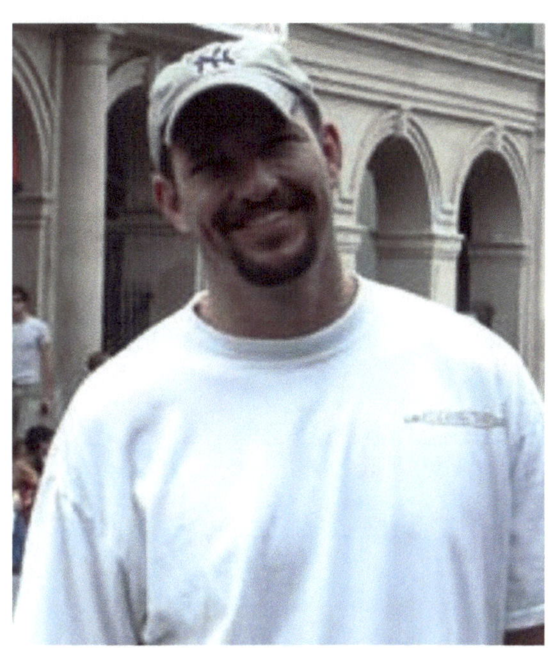

Mark Bingham

When Mark Bingham charged the cockpit,

along with his fellow passengers of Flight 93,

he cemented Cal ruggers' legacy as some of the

most courageous [people in history](). [Robert Paylor]() and [Dominic Cooke](), both former Cal ruggers, have been inspirational in their fight against mobility challenges and have given hope to countless others in similar situations. Dave Nelson, Cal Rugby Class of 1950, uses a walker, but still towers with an impressive frame and a warm smile.

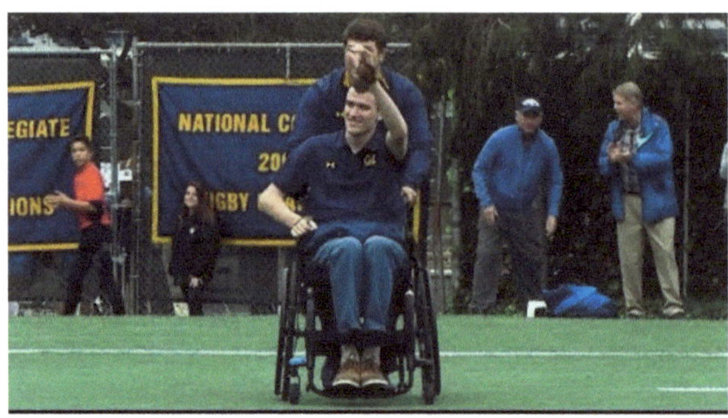

[Robert Paylor]()

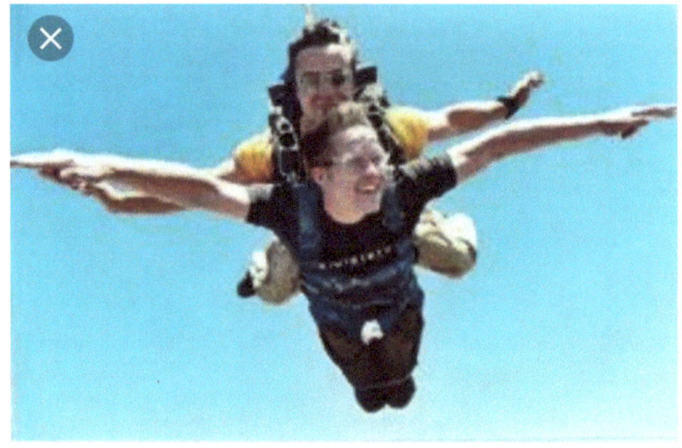

[Dominic Cooke]()

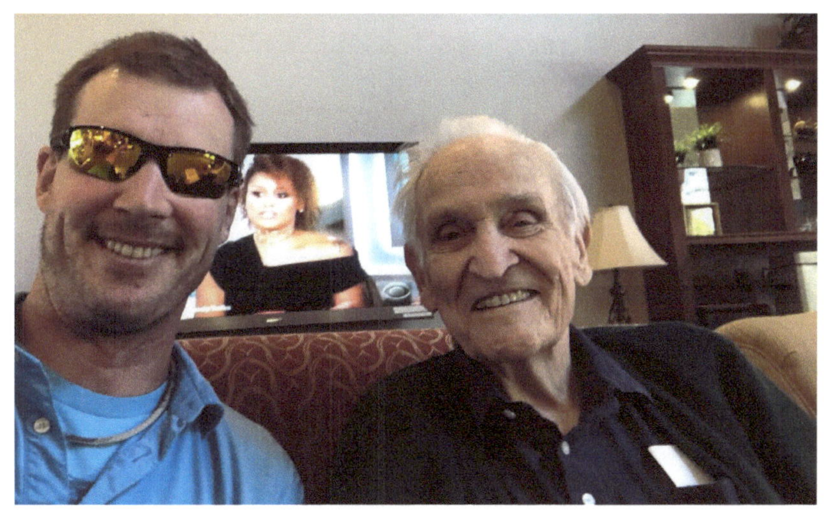

Dan Furlong SMC Rugby 2003 (men's team);

Dave Nelson 1950 Cal Bears Rugby

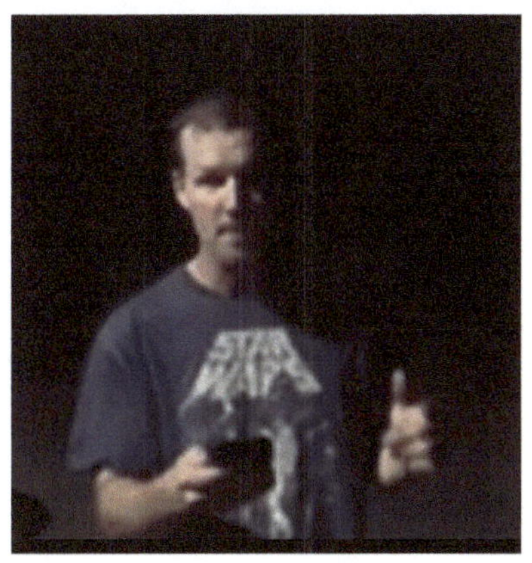

- Learn your rights -

We have been fortunate to have many lawyers who have fought, and are continuing to fight, for the rights of the mobility impaired.

People like David Lepofsky, a blind Canadian lawyer, who was named one of Canada's most influential lawyers in 2010, fight important legal and legislative battles for the mobility impaired.

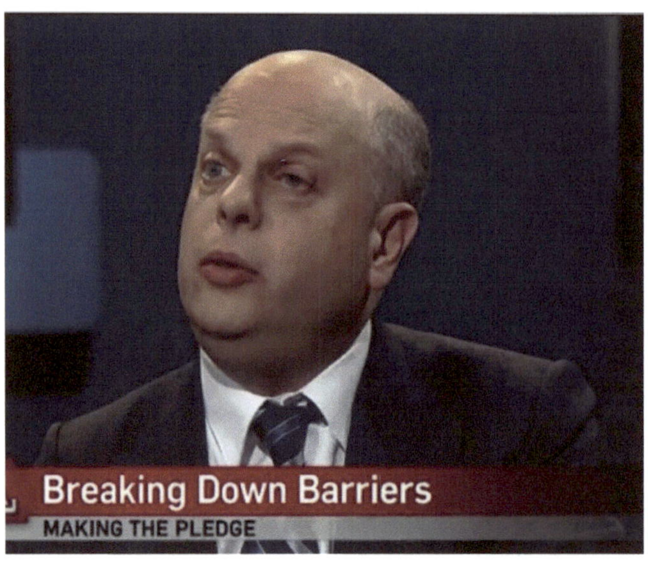

David Lepofsky

- Consider moving to a community supporting a healthy locomotion lifestyle -

There are many great options for those looking to find an engaging and healthy lifestyle. Most of us want to age-in-place and stay mobile. This may require some downsizing, and/or support from a qualified caregiver or loved one.

Find a qualified and trustworthy caregiver, if you think you need one. Also, if you are relocating, search for a trusted realtor whose specialty is working with mobility issues.

The National Aging In Place Council is an excellent resource for information and services for aging-in-place, and has resources for aging-in-place communities. The National Association of Senior Move Managers specializes in helping seniors, and those with mobility challenges, through the downsizing process.

Got Junk? is an excellent resource to assist with downsizing. Silvernest provides cost effective housing options for seniors and those with mobility issues. Life happens quickly, and a good resource for time-sensitive decisions is Caring.com.

You may want to consider finding a trusted caregiver to assist with healthy locomotion. After witnessing his family's struggles finding and managing care for his sister with MS and his uncle who had ALS, Sherwin Sheik founded CareLinx. This platform helps families manage caregiving through web and mobile solutions. Aging-in-place is getting easier and safer because of companies like CareLinx and Envoy.

Envoy is a web based service that assists seniors, and the mobility impaired, and their families by coordinating visits, handyman services, and tech support. Mom's Meals provides fully prepared and refrigerated meals to homes nationwide.

- Use technology to help you move -

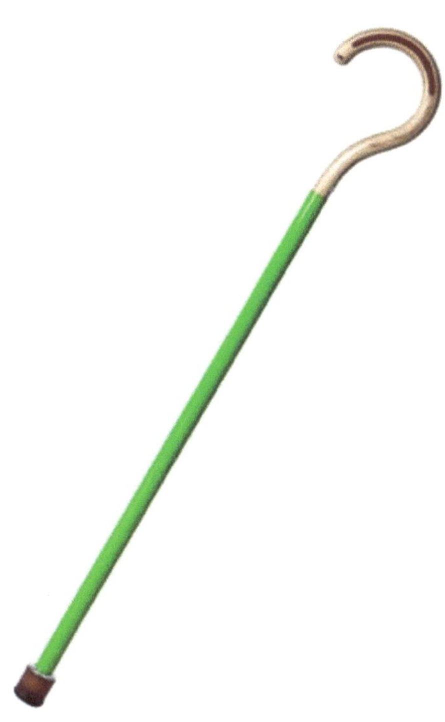

OMHU CANE

Mobility, and senior, focused designers like [Rie Nørregaard](), creator of the Omhu cane, have recently been featured in the [Cooper-Hewitt, Smithsonian Design Museum](). Walkers are also seeing exciting innovations. The [Lifewalker]() upright walker is intelligently designed to help the user feel more confident and aware of their surroundings.

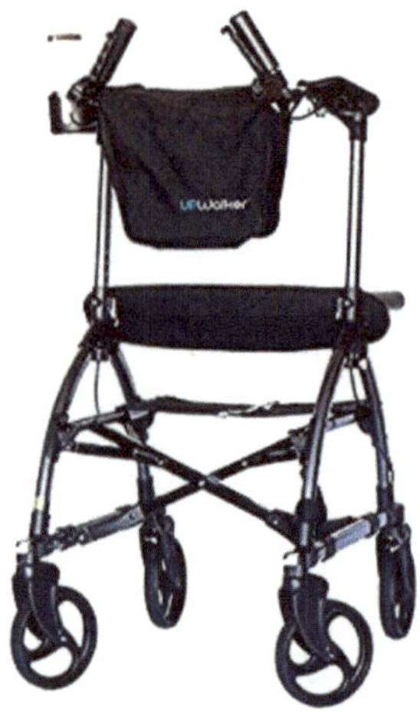

[The Alternative Limb Project](), founded by Sophie Oliveira Barata is on the frontier of innovation in prosthetics. The project is using art and technology to create incredible limbs, hands and feet, that are technologically revolutionary, beautiful, and reflective of the user's personality.

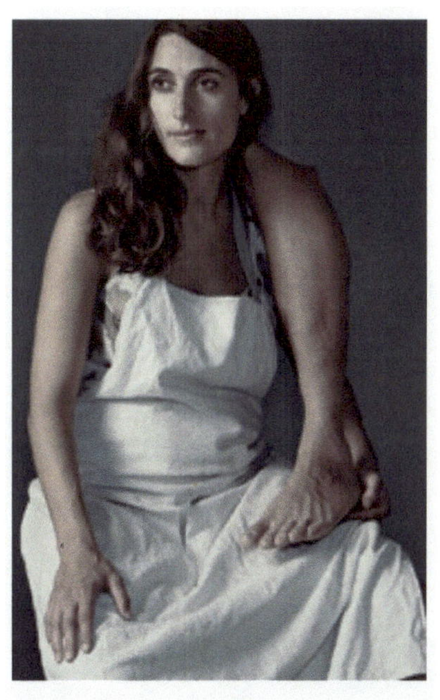

[Sophie Oliveira Barata](#)

The best locomotion technology is seamless and user-friendly. Designers are innovating to the needs of the senior and mobility impaired markets. [Ageless Innovation](#)

is providing engagement for all through user-interactive puppies and kittens.

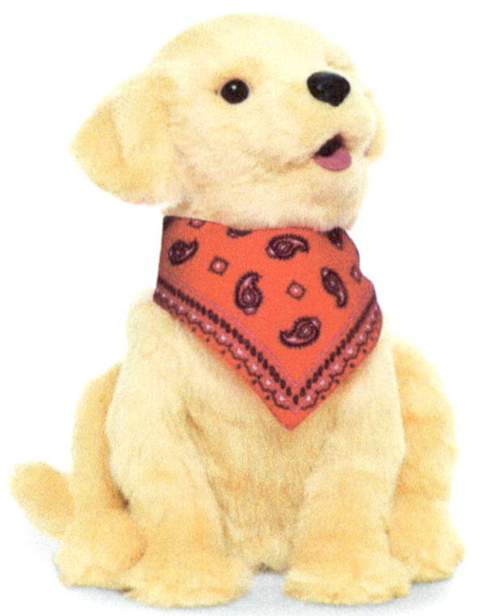

Ageless Innovation Golden Pup

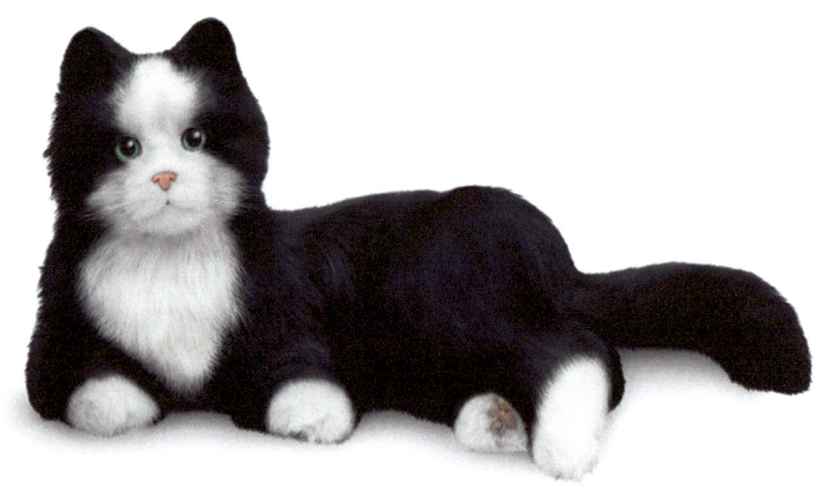

Ageless Innovation Tuxedo Cat

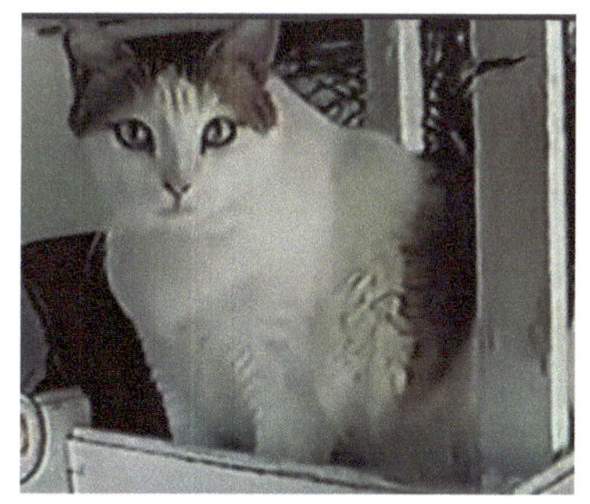

These mess-free pets are a perfect option for seniors and those with mobility issues who have difficulty caring for pets. It has been a joy to see my aunt and her fellow Benedictine [nuns](#) in Bristow, Virginia, enjoy countless hours with their robotic pets. These incredible robotic companions fight loneliness and bring hours of intergenerational joy and play. This simple-to-use, intuitive, technology can brighten the life of anyone who is lonely.

The word technology can be intimidating to some. However, using life changing technology can be as simple as putting on a vest. Cindy Horn of [BalanceWear](#) has created a vest that has restored balance and mobility to those suffering from a wide variety of neurologic and orthopedic disorders such as: MS, Parkinson's, Ataxia, Stroke, Spinal Stenosis, and others.

BalanceWear® Classic Model BW300

There are [systems](#) to keep you safe and systems to help you age in place. [Breezie](#) has designed an easy to use tablet especially for seniors and those with mobility impairments. [Marvee](#) uses [Amazon Device](#) technology to work wonders for caregivers and those looking to age in place and stay mobile.

Getting out and enjoying life is important, especially if you don't drive! There are qualified drivers waiting to pick you up now. Jeff Maltz, CEO of SilverRide, has created a company empowering older adults through mobility, social planning, and a network of caring, friendly drivers putting your safety first.

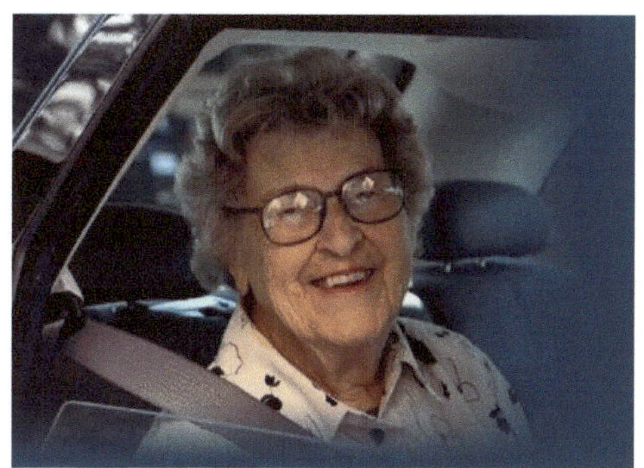

SilverRide

Tesla has been a catalyst for innovation in the auto industry. Their revolutionary thinking in product design is continuing to create a safer and more accessible user experience for all. The engineers at Tesla, Uber, Waymo, GM, Honda, Mercedez-Benz, and many others are creating exciting safety solutions and bringing driverless cars sooner than we can imagine.

New technology is also bridging the gap between cars and non-motorized transport. The miniaturization of the electric motor, battery, and microchip; combined with the utilization of lightweight construction materials such as carbon fiber, and technology such as smart cars and homes, LED, GPS, and Cellular and WiFi data are being leveraged to create products that make mobility easier safer and more fun.

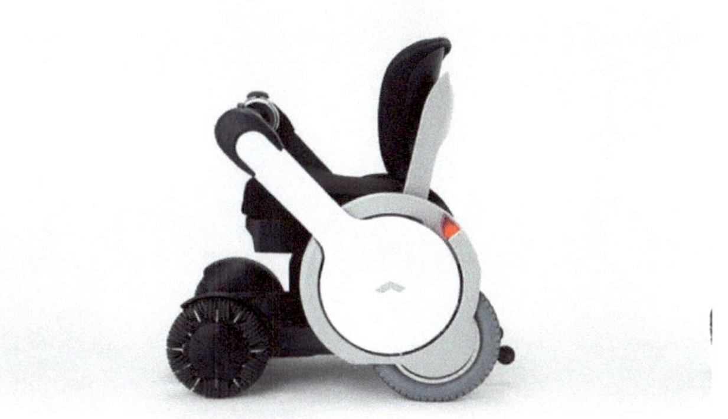

[WHILL Model A](#)

[Wheelchairs](#) and [mobility scooters](#) are moving closer to a designed-for-all concept; transforming from a mobility aid into universal personal transportation. Some mobility scooters, like the [WHILL Model Ci](#), are small enough to fit in the trunk of a car. Wheelchairs like the [Viking 4x4](#) can take you places you never thought possible.

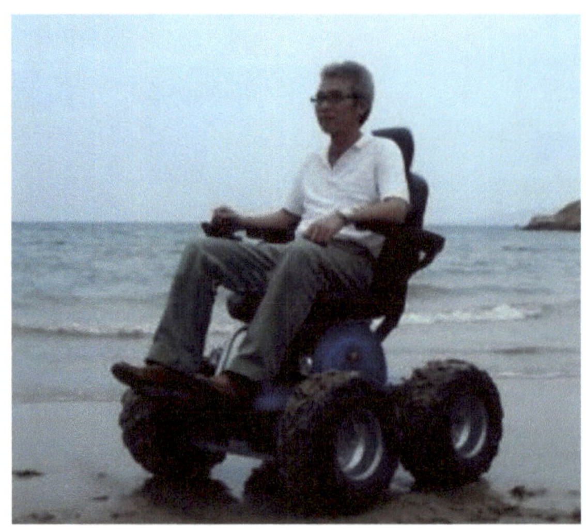

Scooters, ebikes, and trikes are allowing those who have been unable to ride a scooter, bike or trike because of physical impairment an electric boost.

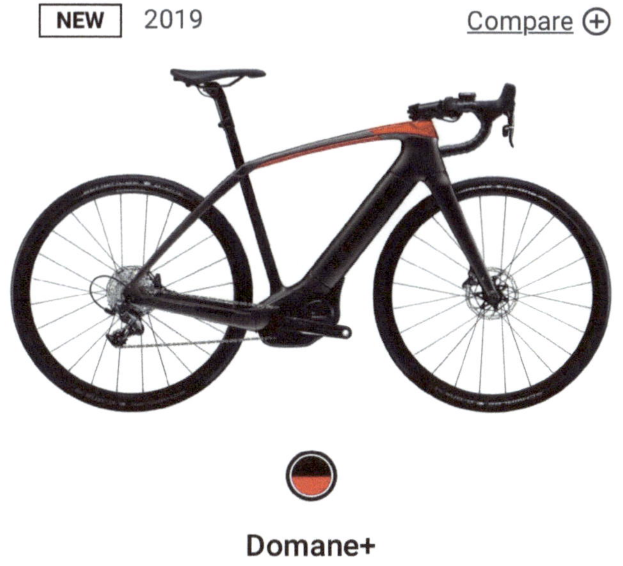

Trek Domane +

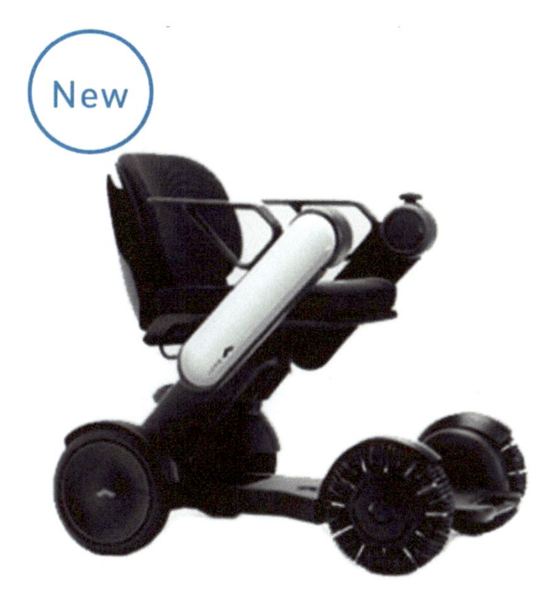

Model Ci | WHILL

Invacare Top End 1195369 Preliminator 10" Seat width
Gecko Green Mini Stock Racing Chair

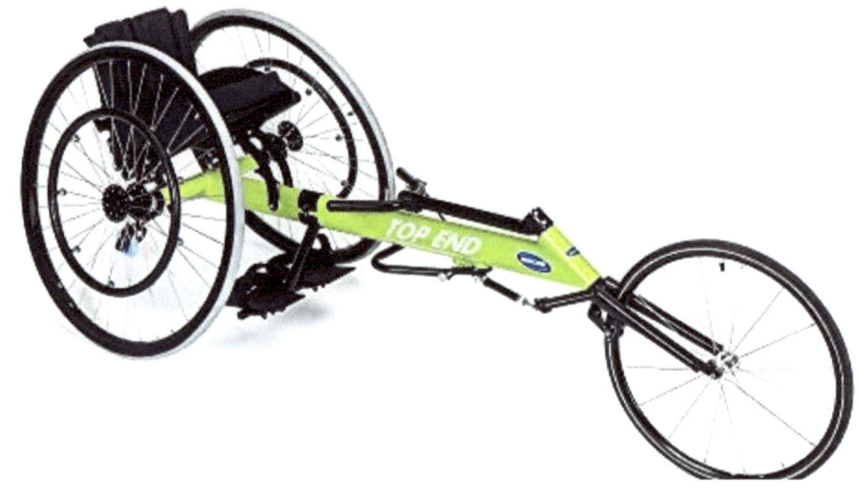

Racing wheelchairs and handcycles are allowing athletes to crush barriers and achieve their goals.

Vans and Recreational Vehicles are great options for those who have mobility impairments.

Ability Equipped

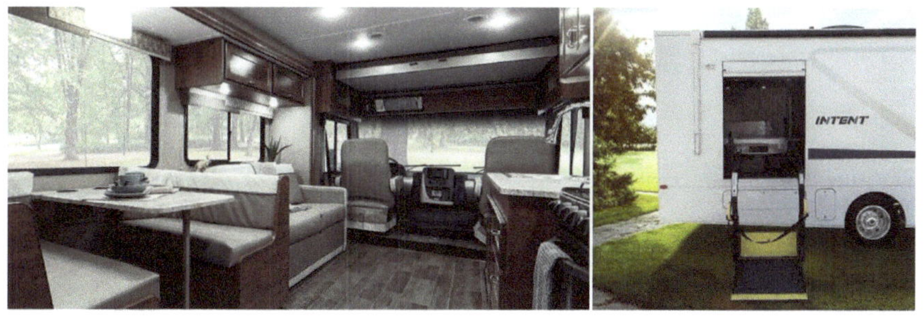

Ability Equipped

Winnebago Industries is pleased to be one of the only RV manufacturers to build motorhomes specifically tailored for those individuals with physical ...

Those with mobility impairments are being helped by innovators like Carrie Shaw, CEO of Embodied Labs, a company that is utilizing VR technology to train caregivers to better understand and care for patients with Alzheimer's and other age, and mobility, related illnesses. Yves Béhar, has designed the superflex aura power suit that improves the user's strength and mobility. Serge Soudoplatoff, his partner Mandy Salomon, and their team at Mentia, have created Deva World for caregivers and patients to play together in a virtual environment.

In the Bay Area, people like Dr. Aaron McPherson of the Center for Elder's Independence are revolutionizing the way we think about aging-in-place and mobility. Insightful and innovative Canadian entrepreneurs like Jeremy Dabor are creating exciting companies in the field of aging and mobility impairment. Important work, yielding incredible results, is also being done with seniors, the mobility impaired, and horses.

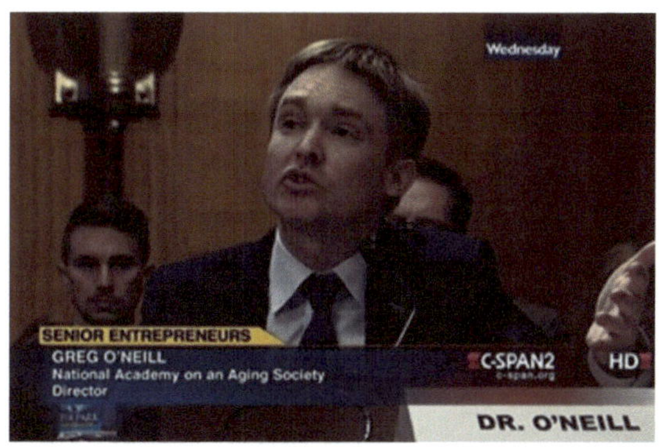

[Dr. Greg O'Neill](#)
1967-2018

Falls are a leading cause of morbidity and mortality in seniors, resulting in tragedy and high costs for insurers. Compounding the issue with falls is the time spent before treatment. There have been several efforts to combat these problems. Researchers at Berkeley's AI Lab have created [fall prevention solutions for memory-care facilities](#) that have reduced falls by 80% with a system called [Safely-You. Fallsafetyapp](#) utilizes technology in your smartphone to detect falls and alert emergency contacts and authorities by text, voice, email, and provides GPS location information.

Laurie Orlov, a highly respected aging and technology analyst, has a [blog](#) with a wise and fair perspective on the technology available to help you age-in-place and stay mobile.

[BestBuy](#) offers excellent training in addressing the needs of seniors, and those with mobility impairments, to its expert sales professionals.

[GreatCall](#) is a leader in providing easy to use healthy locomotion-focused tech like the Jitterbug phone, and 5Star to help you stay connected, in control, and safe.

Tech can even soothe us, [Myndvr](#) is creating Virtual Reality solutions to help seniors and veterans create calming, happy experiences through VR technology.

Intuition Robotics has created the ELLI-Q, an AI driven social robot, designed to engage the user and make it simple to connect with loved ones.

- Appreciate your body -

Treat your body with the respect it deserves. Educate yourself about food. Try and eat good proteins, veggies and fruits, good fats, and watch your electrolyte balance, blood sugar, and cholesterol levels. Calculate your BMR and your BMI. Learn about the importance of calcium and fiber to build strong bones and facilitate healthy digestion.

Learn about your body's systems and what you can do to to help them healthier. Educate yourself about supplements. See your doctor, and ask about procedures and medications that can increase longevity and decrease morbidity. Secure your electronic documentation for advance care planning.

Learn your genetic profile to understand your cultural background and possible predisposition for disease. There is exciting work done by Ping Zhang and his team at Jintel Health using "intelligence as a service" to combat disease.

Be sure to ask your medical professional about protein, vitamins, minerals, and other nutrition in your diet, as well as supplements like glucosamine-chondroitin-MSM, resveratrol, antioxidants, fish oil, pharmaceuticals, etc. Ask what he or she thinks might be good ideas for you add to your health regimen. Learn about the exciting research being conducted on extending our lifespan and preventing the diseases associated with aging, and mobility issues.

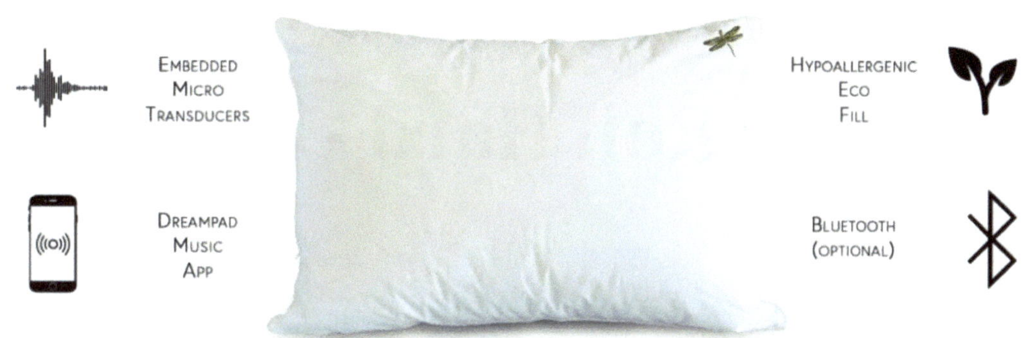

Dreampad

Practice good hygiene; sleep and otherwise. You may also want to consider medical marijuana, or other alternative therapies. Give yourself credit for empowering yourself and deciding to take control on your healthy locomotion journey.

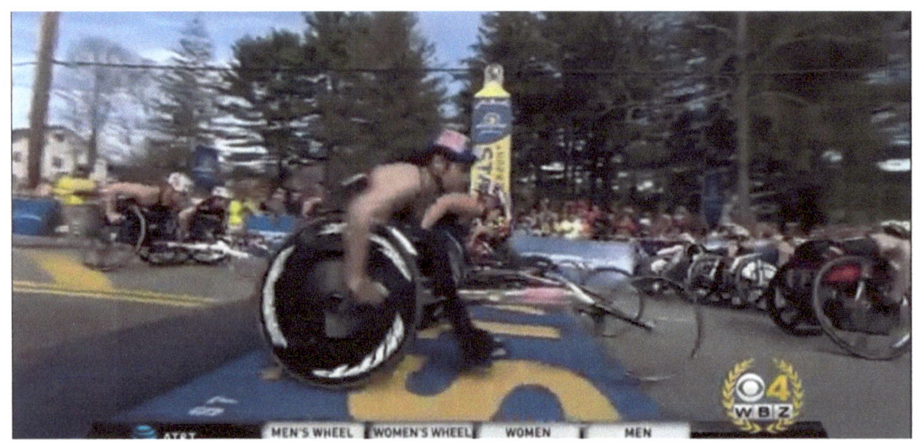

- Roll Hard -

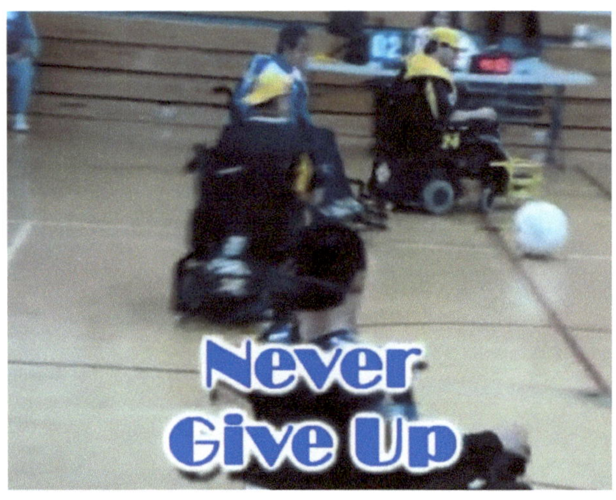

- Glendale Rough Riders -

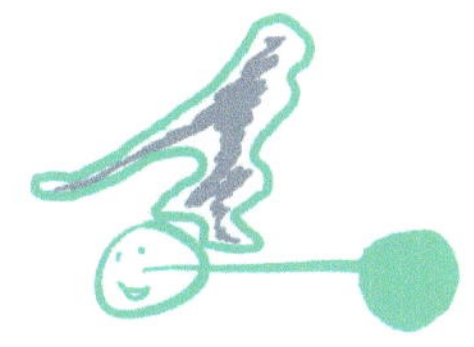

- **The Rocklocomotion Menu** -

Museums

The Archway
The Disability History Museum
The Broad
The Huntington Library
Monticello
Mount Vernon
The Getty
British Museum
The Palace Museum
Goethe House
Imperial War Museum
The Queensland Museum
Melbourne Museum
Royal Exhibition Building (Melbourne)
Australian Museum

Pacific Aviation Museum
9/11 Memorial
Van Gogh Museum
Museum of Alchemists & Magicians of Old Prague
Museum of Mummies of Guanajuato
National Museum of Anthropology (Mexico)
Prison Gate Museum (Netherlands)
Styrian Armory Museum (Austria)
Vasa Museum (Sweden)
Viking Ship Museum (Norway)
Whitney Plantation
Messner Mountain Museum (Italy)
Sarawak State Museum (Malaysia)
Smithsonian Institution
Arcade Museum
Belgian Brewer's Museum
Burlesque Hall of Fame
Coffee Museum (Brazil)
Erawan Museum (Thailand)
Ghibli Museum (Japan)
Grammy Museum
The Green Vault
The Taj Mahal
Museum of Childhood
Museum of Childhood (Edinburgh)
Charles Schultz Museum

Norton Simon Museum
De Young Museum
Academy of Sciences
Exploratorium
Lawrence Hall of Science
Field Museum
Musical Instruments Museum
Soumaya Museum
Vodka Museum
Bicycle Museum of America
Big Hole and Open Mine Museum
National Maritime Museum (France)
National Rail Museum (U.K.)
New Mexico Museum of Space History
New York City Fire Museum
Porsche Museum
The Ferrari Museum
The Henry Ford Museum of American Innovation
GM Heritage Center
Allpar Museum
Toyota Museum
Mercedes Museum
B.M.W. Museum
Gopher Hole Museum
Watermelon Museum (China)
Clown Hall of Fame and Research Center

[Jelly Belly Factory](#)
[Cupnoodles Museum](#)
[Budweiser Brewery Tours](#)
[Coors Brewery Tours](#)
[Anchor Steam Brewery](#)
[Sulabh Museum of Toilets](#)

Movies

[African Queen](#)
[Me Before You](#)
[Murderball](#)
[Rise and Walk: The Dennis Byrd Story](#)
[Blues Brothers](#)
[Casablanca](#)
[Singing in the Rain](#)
[To Kill a Mockingbird](#)
[As Good as it Gets](#)
[Back to School](#)
[Rocky Balboa](#)
[Cleopatra](#)
[Patch Adams](#)
[Batteries Not Included](#)
[Cocoon](#)
[Blue Hawaii](#)

[Driving Miss Daisy](#)
[The Shawshank Redemption](#)
[Awakenings](#)
[Forrest Gump](#)
[Smokey and the Bandit](#)
[Life is Beautiful](#)
[Don Juan DeMarco](#)

Community & Rights

[U.S. Dept of Justice Disability Rights](#)
[Department of Justice Elder Abuse Resources](#)
[United States Fire Administration Elder Safety](#)
[United States Equal Opportunity Employment Commission](#)
[WHO](#)
[AARP](#)
[AARP Foundation](#)
[AARP (en español)](#)
[AARP Foundation Litigation](#)
[Sparkpeople](#)
[SilverSneakers](#)
[Seniornet](#)
[Startsat60](#)
[Gerontological Society](#)
[ASA](#)

NCOA
National Alliance on Caregiving
SeniorCorps
Kupunawiki
Habitat for Humanity

Health, Wellness, Cognitive Fitness

SilverSneakers
Sparkpeople
Orangetheoryfitness
24hourFitness
PositScience
SingFit
GNC
WebMD
Gerontological Society
HealthCare
VyncaHealth
Kaiser
United Healthcare
OctaviaWellness
Linkage
TripleTree
Active Daily Living

Jintel Health
Masterpiece Living
Next Avenue

Employment

WAHVE
SeniorLiving

Legal and Financial Services

FirstRepublic
EverSafe
LifeSite
BankSafe
Ziegler
MidOceanPartners
American Bar Association
California Bar Association
Los Angeles Bar Association
National Association of Financial Advisors
Professional Fiduciary Association of California
National Association of Certified Financial Fiduciaries

Rocketlawyer
Legalzoom

Technology Solutions

EmbodiedLabs
PositScience
ThinOptics
GreatCall
BestBuy
MyndVR
Elliq
Ohmni Labs
SingFit
EverSound
Ageless Innovation
On the Muv
Comcast
Marvee
Breezie
It's Never Too Late
Bluestar SeniorTech
Mentia

SafelyYou
CDW
Cabhi
CITRIS
Got Junk?
Dreampad
MPTF

Fall Prevention and Mobility Technology

FallSafetyApp
SafelyYou
Omhu Cane
LifeWalker
Drive Medical Spitfire Scout Scooter
Pride Jazzy Zero Turn Scooter
Segway

Caregiving

Envoy
LivPact
Carelinx
GreatCall Family Caregiving Solutions

TheMemoryKit
ComfortKeepers
Vyncahealth
Home Care Assistance

Transportation

SilverRide
Uber
Lyft
Quantas
Tesla

Entertainment, Fun & Travel

Getty Images
SilverRide
Playstation
Oculus Rift
Nintendo
Xbox
Hagerty
Barrett Jackson Auctions

Mecum Auctions
GolfNow
Fandango
Stubhub
Viking River Cruises
Carnival Cruise Line
SingFit
LonelyPlanet
Pandora
Tesla
YouTube

Retail

Amazon
BestBuy
First Street
SeniorBlueBook

People: John Williams, David Inns, Jo Ann Jenkins, Norman Lear, Jack Lalanne, Jane Glenn Haas, Gail Sheehy, Mary Furlong, Oprah Winfrey, Elon Musk, Hubert Joley, Carrie Shaw, Laurie Orlov, Lori Bitter, Jeff Maltz, Ken Dychwald, Jody Holtzman, Paul Irving, Guy Kawasaki, Katy Fike, Sherri Snelling, Paul Kleyman, David Lindeman, Jeh Kazimi, Robert

Blancato, Michael Carroll, John Hopper, Scott Smith, Dr. Sanjaya Kumar, Jeremy Dabor, Dr. Aaron K. McPherson, Ping Zhang, Sherwin Sheik, Ted Fischer, Saeko Tsuchihashi

Books: Turning Silver into Gold by Mary Furlong, AgeWave by Ken Dychwald, A Cast of Caregivers by Sherri Snelling, Disrupt Aging by Jo Ann Jenkins, Even This I Get To Experience by Norman Lear, Still Foolin' 'Em: Where I've been, Where I'm going, and Where the Hell are my Keys by Billy Crystal, Parkinson's Treatment: 10 Secrets to a Happier Life by Michael S. Okun M.D., Measure What Matters by John Doerr, The Longevity Economy: Unlocking the World's Fastest-Growing, Most Misunderstood Market, by Joseph F. Coughlin, Passages by Gail Sheehy, A Bittersweet Season by Jane Gross, Being Mortal by Atul Gawande, Can't We Talk About Something More Pleasant by Roz Chast, The Complete Eldercare Planner by Joy Loverde, A Pirate Looks at 50 by Jimmy Buffett, The Telomere Effect by Dr's Elizabeth Blackburn & Elissa Epel, The Longevity Plan: 7 Life Transforming Lessons From Ancient China by John D. Day M.D., In Defense of Food by Michael Pollan, The Heart of the Plate: Vegetarian Recipes for a New Generation by Molly Katzen, The Silverado Story: A Memorycare Culture

[Where Love is Greater Than Fear](#) by Loren Shook and Stephen Winner, [Stumbling on Happiness](#) by Daniel Gilbert, [I Feel Bad About My Neck: and other thoughts on being a woman](#) by Nora Ephron, [The Woman Who Changed Her Brain: How I Left my Learning Disability Behind and Other Stories of Cognitive Transformation](#) by Barbara Arrowsmith-Young, [Never Split The Difference: Negotiating As If Your Life Depended On It](#) by Christopher Voss, [The Undoing Project](#) by Michael Lewis, [Coach: Lessons on the Game of Life](#) by Michael Lewis, [Values of the Game](#) by Bill Bradley, [Blue Highways](#) by William Least-Heat Moon, [The Joy of Living](#) by Eric Swanson and Yongey Mingyur Rinpoche, [100 Plus: How the Coming Age of Longevity Will Change Everything](#) by Sonia Arrison, [Flow: The Psychology of Optimal Experience](#) by Mihaly Csikszentmihalyi